How and Where to Buy Rich CBD Oil Online

The Complete Guide on buying rich CBD Oil online safely

Ashley M. Wadsworth

Copyright © 2018 by Ashley M. Wadsworth

All rights reserved. No part of this publication may be reproduced, distributed, or transmitted in any form or by any means, including photocopying, recording, or other electronic or mechanical methods, without the prior written permission of the publisher, except in the case of brief quotations embodied in critical reviews and certain other non-commercial uses permitted by copyright law.

Copyright © Ashley M. Wadsworth

Dedication

This book is dedicated to all who desire to purchase quality and rich CBD Oil.

Table of Contents

How and Where to Buy Rich CBD Oil Online 1

Dedication 3

Introduction 7

Chapter 1 10

    The CBD Oil 10

    Can CBD Oil get me Intoxicated? 12

    Side Effects of CBD 13

Chapter 2 17

    Uses of CBD Oil 17

        CBD oil is a Medicine 17

    Is CBD oil safe to Use? 18

Chapter 3 19

    How does Cannabidiol (CBD) work inside one's body? 19

    How do I buy the CBD Oil? 20

Chapter 4 22

Great Tips and Tricks to buy CBD oil 22

Conclusion 31

About The Author 33

Disclaimer 34

Acknowledgement 35

PAGE LEFT INTENTIONALLY

Introduction

Thank you for taking the time to download this book: How and Where to Buy Rich CBD OIL Online - The Complete Guide on buying rich CBD Oil online safely.

This book covers the topic of CBD, its uses and tips on how to buy the CBD Oil safely online.

The plant Cannabis sativa has been used in medicinal practice for thousands of years.

In this book, you will learn exactly what CBD and hemp oil is and how it can benefit you...

- Manage physical pain

- Enhance your mood

- Increase your memory

- Help your immune system

- Act as aphrodisiac

- Control your appetite

- Help you sleep

- Clear your skin

- Strengthen your heart

And lots more,

This book will take you from knowing nothing about CBD to being an expert in no time.

Cannabis is a complex plant with more than 400 chemical entities of which over 60 of them are cannabinoid compounds, some of them with opposing effects.

At the completion of this book, you will have a good understanding of CBD oil and be able to use them responsibly to get out its full health benefits

Once again, thank you for purchasing this book. I hope you find it to be helpful.

Chapter 1

The CBD Oil

CBD oil is a botanical oil produced from the seeds and stalks of the cannabis plants. These plants are naturally rich in CBD and contain a low THC. It has a specialised technique used to extract the CBD oil and it contains nutritious elements such as vitamins, terpenes, omega-three fatty acids, minerals, amino acids and chlorophyll.

The CBD hemp oil is seen in most health food stores and markets. The hemp oil is obtained from the hemp seed containing only trace volume of CBD. The products of hemp seed contains very low quantity of CBD with regards to weight which makes them insufficient for those who seek to balance the CBD effect.

The need for CBD hemp oil has increased in the recent years making the market to respond by coming up with new and different types of products of CBD oil. There are varieties of CBD hemp oil product in the market.

Natural and pure CBD oil that can be used on their own are now available in drops, tablets, tinctures, drinks, and chewing gum.

If you are one of those who avoid trace amounts of THC seen in almost all the products of CBD hemp oil, then, the no amount-THC of CBD hemp oil products are now available in many stores and markets recently.

Can CBD Oil get me Intoxicated?

The major question asked by users of cannabidiol (CBD) is about its compound properties and to know about the benefits of taking CBD oil. Users really want to know if taking or using the CBD oil will intoxicate them.

The shortest answer to this question is a capital NO! CBD oil cannot get any one high. CBD oil is hauled out from cannabis plant.

A common fallacy is that it will bring out a euphoric result, but the basic truth is that, CBD oil is absolutely non-psychoactive, and does not in any way have an adverse effect on attention, behaviour, perception or sensory cognizance.

CBD oil has no extra trace quantity of (THC) tetrahydrocannabinol, which happens to be the psychoactive cannabinoid that provokes the "dim" or "stoned" mind-changing feelings which might be generally related to the use of marijuana. CBD oil is taken out from the seeds and stalks of hemp that contains only about 0.3 percent of THC per dry weight, or thirty-three times lower than the least powerful euphoric-initiating cannabis strain.

Rather, the CBD oil contains a whole lot of CBD, which has proven to have the competence to counter the psychoactive properties of THC.

Side Effects of CBD

The side effects of CBD are:

1. **Low Blood pressure**

High dosage of CBD oil daily may cause a minimum drop in blood pressure. This drop in blood pressure is often connected with feelings of light-headedness. This side effect is temporary and can be mitigated by drinking a cup of tea or coffee.

2. **Drowsiness or Wakefulness**

CBD can cause drowsiness when high dose is consumed. If this is the way you feel when you ingest CBD, it is safe not to drive a vehicle or operate any machine equipment.

In most cases however, CBD serves as a wake-inducing agent.

3. **Dry mouth**

The commonly described side effect of the administration of CBD is the dry sensation it causes within the mouth. This appears to be caused by the connection of the endocannabinoid system in inhibiting saliva secretion. This effect may be mitigated by drinking a glass of water.

4. **Increased quiver in Parkinson's disease when high dose CBD is consumed.**

Research carried out by some group of scientists confirms that high doses of CBD may worsen muscle movement in individuals that suffers from Parkinson's disease. Other studies also recommend cannabidiol to be safe and well tolerable by patients of Parkinson's disease.

In this case, reducing CBD dose intake will reduce this possible side effect. Sufferers of Parkinson's disease should consult with their doctor before consuming CBD and should start by taking smaller doses.

5. Inhibition of hepatic drug metabolism

CBD can interact with specific series of pharmaceutical drugs because it has been proven to inhibit cytochrome p450, a group of liver enzymes responsible for the breaking down of an extensive range of pharmaceutical medicines. If a high dose of CBD is ingested, the cannabinoid can temporarily neutralize the activity of p450 enzymes, thus changing the way drugs are metabolized inside the body. The effect is however minor.

If you're currently using pharmaceutical drugs and still interested in consuming CBD, discuss with your doctor or pharmacist.

Chapter 2

Uses of CBD Oil

CBD oil is a Medicine

CBD oil is a medicine used in treating many health conditions such as:

1. Nausea and vomiting.
2. Anxiety
3. Bone growth
4. Nervous system degeneration
5. Chronic pain
6. Cancer cell growth
7. Insomnia
8. Low appetite
9. Bacteria growth
10. High blood sugar

11. Muscle spasms

12. Artery blockage

13. Inflammation

14. Seizures and convulsions

15. Psychoses

16. Psoriasis

Is CBD oil safe to Use?

Many that are curious about beginning with CBD oil do worry about the safety of using this product. They usually want to know if it will get high and if it's safe to use around kids.

Thankfully, CBD does not cause harm because it is non-psychoactive and has minimal side effects.

Chapter 3

How does Cannabidiol (CBD) work inside one's body?

CBD is the core active ingredient in hemp and unlike Tetrahydrocannabinol (THC), it is not psychoactive, therefore, it does not get a person intoxicated. The body system of human comprises of endocannabinoid system and receptors spread through the body and brain. THC triggers two receptors (CB1 and CB2), while CBD does not exactly stimulate any of these receptors; it rather stimulates other receptors like adenosine, serotonin receptors and vanilloid.

How do I buy the CBD Oil?

The CBD oil is generally available in recent times due to the constant research and studies which have proved its efficacy. It is now made legal in the world because of its non-psychoactive effects, though, it can be a daunting task to get reliable CBD product.

You are to pay adequate attention when searching for quality CBD products so as to purchase the original CBD product.

Many people mix up CBD oil for THC (the ingredient found in cannabis which is responsible for the psychoactive effects that leads to having a high feeling and this has resulted into different mixed opinions and reviews about the CBD product. Many people still perceive CBD oil to be a drug that provides a high feeling effect due to its association with cannabis.

However, laboratory and clinical tests has proven that CBD oil can't and will not get the user intoxicated.

Chapter 4

Great Tips and Tricks to buy CBD oil

These are the simple steps you need to consider to get a high quality and rich CBD oil from online stores. Reliable and trustworthy sellers' keeps their integrity by always providing you with detailed information connected to the product you are purchasing.

1. Search for first-class products rather than the reduced-priced products.

Once you have made the decision to buy CBD oil, go to Google where you will find numerous search results. There are different products readily available in the market place due to the difference in price, extraction methods and quantity.

Keep in mind that getting quality CBD oil can never be low-prices and that is a fact. Many people have chosen low prices over quality and leave negative reviews when the aim of purchasing the CBD oil is not achieved. Bear in mind that if you are aim at getting inexpensive products from the market, it can never be effective.

Many providers of CBD oil and sellers have capitalized on the point that CBD oil is gradually gaining popularity all over the globe due to its health benefit and have decided to profit easily by selling fake products of CBD. Be wise; don't be lured by low prices.

The best way to recognize a high quality CBD product is to request for third-party lab inquiry from the vendor.

Authentic CBD oil providers will feed you with basic information about the product as well as the source and full concentration of cannabidiol.

Check to see the concentration of cannabidiol because the greater the cannabidiol level, the more effective the product will be.

2. CBD volume

Check the CBD volume within the product when buying CBD oil. Since the CBD oils are obtainable in different volumes, you would need to know the quantity of CBD you will be ingesting for every dose taken.

You cannot afford to go on an overdose as you will need to know the amount of CBD oil your body can carry to cure the medical condition.

The CBD oil concentration relies on the fundamental health issues. Therefore, it is best you consult with someone who has used CBD oil already or you strictly adhere to the dosage guide. It is also advisable you begin with a low dose of CBD oil and increase gradually.

3. Volume of hemp seed oil

There are two main components you should be concerned about when you are about to buy the CBD oil.

a. CBD volume

b. Volume of hemp seed oil

The Hemp seed oil volume is the quantity of hemp oil available in the product.

Hemp oil also has its health benefit but you need to be sure of the CBD concentration in the product you are purchasing when buying CBD products. Buying an item with high concentration of hemp oil and a low content of CBD is like taking in fish oil with additional EPA and DHA without the main ingredients.

4. Study the CBD product Label

Some hemp products are sold with psychoactive compounds which results in unpleasant effects. However, the CBD oil is extracted from industrial hemp or food-grade hemp with little or no amount of THC.

So, choose only CBD products with non-psychoactive ingredients as stated on the labels.

5. CBD concentration

The concentration of CBD is all about the amount of CBD present in the whole volume of CBD product. As earlier stated, CBD oil has several other products aside from CBD so bear in mind the amount of CBD present before buying any CBD product.

The permitted dosage for starters is between 2-3gms. However, you can begin with 10 mg depending on your height and weight and adjust accordingly.

To achieve the desired result of this oil, use the product consistently. If you are unable to achieve the desired effect with first dosage, increase your consumption of CBD and observe the result over time.

6. Check the product website for product reviews

The CBD oil industry is still fresh and young. Getting a company with proven track records about the CBD products can be very tough.

When buying your quality CBD products, make sure you are buying products from a vendor of good repute by reading the product reviews on the internet.

7. Customer service

The integrity of the vendors can be quickly accessed by contacting them directly. Reliable and well recognised companies have a good customer service representative that answers all queries concerning a particular purchase.

You can easily get in touch with them via phone, email or live chat. The customer service representative would be glad to provide the answers to all your queries.

8. Manufacturers Identification of where the plant was originated from

The CBD oil can be identified by examining the product to be free from chemical pesticides and herbicides.

The CBD plant should be cultivated on a land where there is no prior refuse dump as the plants can take in contaminants and industrial wastes. These wastes can be deposited into the body once CBD is consumed.

9. Method of Extraction

The procedures of CBD oil extraction have the capacity to cause creation of harmful solvents in traces.

Dependable CBD manufacturers choose an extraction technique that gives the purest type of the CBD oil.

The well known method of extraction used by recognized companies is the Supercritical Fluid Extraction using Carbon dioxide or CO_2 technology.

10. Go for a non - GMO product

Genetically modified organism (GMO) is a modern technology and not much is identified about its effect on the human body. Scientific studies have however reported that GMO's contain toxins, boosts the susceptibility of disease, less nutritious, and might damage the soil which will call for increased application of pesticides.

Conclusion

CBD Oil is the new miracle treatment that treats several health conditions.

The essential nutrient it contains makes it acceptable by all.

Try out the recipes recommended in this book and you will never regret it.

I believe you found this book useful Why not gift it to friends and family to benefit too.

Thank you for reading the book.

THE END

Did you enjoy reading this book? Please remember to leave a positive review. Thank you.

About The Author

Ashley M. Wadsworth is a researcher and a humanitarian

Disclaimer

This book contains information that is intended to help the readers be better informed consumers of health care.

It is presented as general advice on health care.

This book is not intended to be a substitute for the medical advice of a licensed physician. The reader should consult with their doctor in any matters relating to his/her health.

By reading this document, the reader agrees that under no circumstances is the author responsible for any losses, direct or indirect, which are incurred as a result of the use of information contained within this document, including, but not limited to, errors, omissions, or inaccuracies.

Acknowledgement

I thank God for the success of this book.